Mantra Yoga

The Art of Listening, Reciting and Transforming

"EDUCAZIONE VEDICA"
Training Program in Bhakti yoga

www.educazionevedica.org

educazionevedica@gmail.com

INDEX

Introduction

"Powerful Words, Secret Codes, Magical Phrases!"

History shows us how humankind has always given great importance and weight to the power that a simple single word, a sound, a concept, can acquire at a specific time and place. A power capable of altering the energies of Nature and of transforming the destiny of an individual, a community and even entire nations.

I am reminded of that famous magic formula that captivates children when listening to the exotic folk tale of Ali Baba and the Forty Thieves: "Open sesame!" Those two magic words that opened the prodigious door to a cave filled with immense treasures.

In everyday life, we are constantly using words and phrases that can immediately influence our behaviour and the behaviour of others, positively or negatively.

Sometimes we hear **words** and **phrases** that open up for us, even **dramatically**, new **scenarios**, new **inner visions**, new **energy stages** to be probed, hitherto totally **unexpected** and often taking us by **surprise**. Sounds and words that can give us access to **deep** levels of **consciousness**, otherwise **unreachable** in our modest daily lives.

The tradition of using the transformative power of words and sounds is certainly universal. It has been used and studied by all cultures and societies in the universe.

In the next chapters we will explore how the VEDAs, the ancient writings of the VEDIC CULTURE, presented and used the power of speech through the sacred sounds of the **VEDIC MANTRAs**.

What is special about the **VEDIC CULTURE** is that it developed the art of **sacred sounds** into a perfect, exact, **science** in which the **MANTRA** uses the power of sound and speech to be able to experience a sacred approach to the **integrated vision** of **life** and **consciousness** (matter and spirit).

In other words, the **MANTRA** is the **tool** to be able to **reach** higher and higher stages of **consciousness**, from more basic earthly energy levels to levels of great spiritual intensity.

The word **MANTRA** has now entered common language and many people use it to mean a **'magic formula,'** a **'spell'** that has some subliminal effect at a deep level. Most likely this is because it has been understood that the vast majority of

fears and **inner blocks** that prevent us from being truly happy are hidden in the unconscious mind.

But in reality, the use of VEDIC MANTRAs is a science that works on multiple levels.

Therefore there is an increasing interest in knowing how to best use the power of **VEDIC MANTRAs** to improve one's life, generate and/or recover **prosperity**, **physical** and **mental well**-**being**, have **better** social **relationships**, or simply for **personal** and **spiritual growth**.

In addition to understanding what the Vedic Mantras are and how they work, what do we offer that is special in this book?

We will try to study, explore and connect with '**personal**' mantras, i.e., those mantras that do not only refer to a concept of energy, but will allow you to connect with the '**Person**', the '**Character** of the **Mantra**', with His/Her specific **Nature** and **Qualities**.

We will access this '**personal aspect**' together through some unique and exclusive **stories, tales,** that will enable you to sublimate the effects of reciting the MANTRAs.

The Word, the Sound, the Vibration

Each Word has two intrinsic elements: **Sound** and **Meaning**.

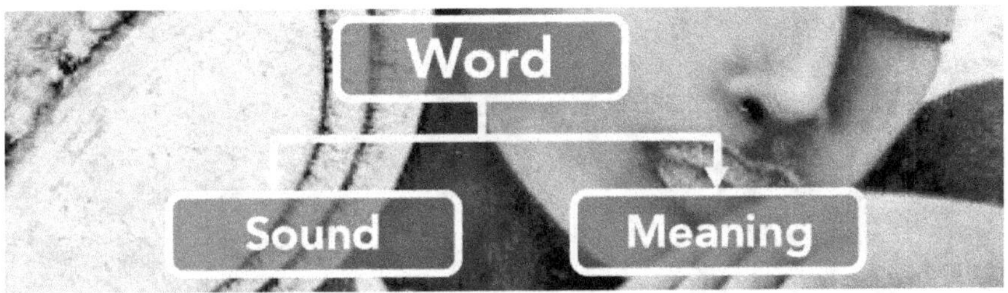

Sound represents the element that **conveys** Meaning.

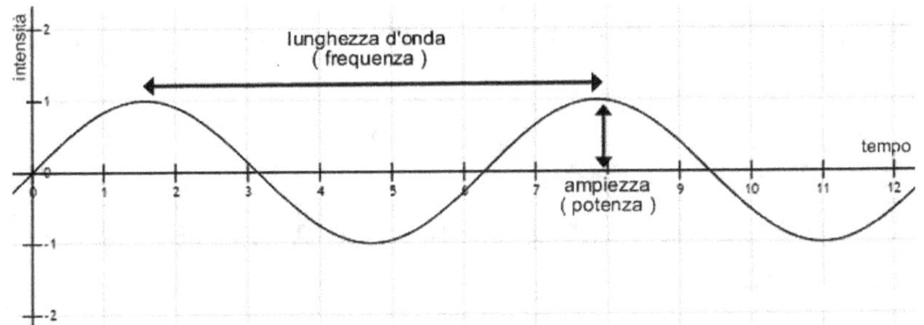

How does this process take place?

The Word is Sound, and Sound is Vibration that propagates in the air as a longitudinal wave with a certain direction of propagation and is also characterised by a precise **frequency** and **power** (amplitude).

When we utter a word, for example the term 'Love,' the **sound**, as a vibration, **will transfer the meaning and energy of the word to the receptive object**.

Is it possible that a sound wave with specific frequency can energetically interact with elements and particles of matter?

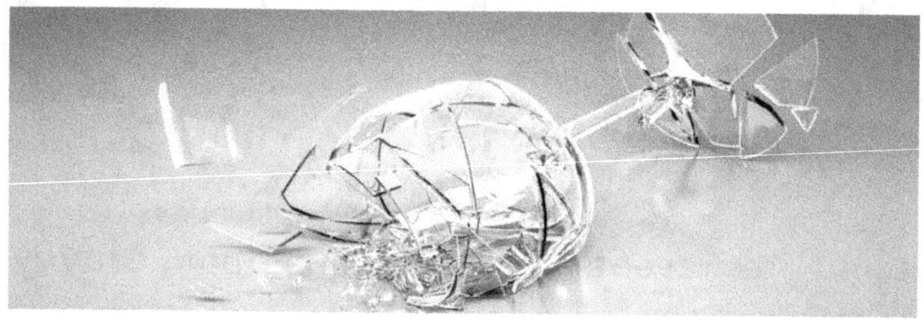

We all experience this on a daily basis, but I would like to bring you some obvious examples and applications.

The most classic example of how a sound vibration can interact with a physical object is the case of a specific musical note that brings to a **state of resonance**, and thus **breakage**, an element of particular structural hardness and fragility, such as the classic crystal glass, that at a certain moment shatters.

How does the **glass shatter**?

In simple words, a vibration (singer's voice) can create a sound with a frequency similar to the frequency of the invested system (the glass).

Consequently, a **resonance** phenomenon is triggered that leads to a significant **energy buildup** within the stressed system, which, in specific cases, leads to rupture (energy release).

Another example of interaction between sound and matter is the invasive effect of excessive exposure to very loud, protracted noise (sounds) on the human being's auditory system resulting in damage to the auditory receptive organ.

Most of us live in urban environments and experience daily the disturbance caused by traffic, neighbours, and so on, and we experience on our skin the consequences on the auditory system and also on our psychic apparatus (nervousness, stress, headaches).

The examples we have cited imply a broader view of matter, namely that every **object** in the **cosmos** is 'phaEnergy'.

If we accept this **energetic conception of matter**, then, every chemical element, every cell, every organ in the human body, every **structure** in the **universe** is **oscillating energy**.

Energy is vibration, which is characterised by precise oscillating frequency.

Quantum Physics itself bases its assumptions and theses on considering that every **element** and object of matter **fluctuates**, oscillates (i.e., has a frequency). In other words, **that** it is **Energy**.

Where do these observations lead to?

To the conclusion that **Words**, **Sounds**, and specifically **MANTRAs**, have the **ability** to **interrelate**, interact, with all **material elements** and **enable us to reach and activate different levels of energy**.

The **crucial factor** that activates these exchanges is the **interaction** between **frequencies**.

According to the research of Masaru Emoto, an independent Japanese researcher, the **water** element has the special property of 'registering' the positive and negative **psychic stimuli** it receives from the environment in the form of **sound** (manifest or non-manifest). Then **water changes** its **structure (water memory)**.

How can one not wonder, then, what the **effects** of these same stimuli -- **thoughts, words, emotions,**

sounds -- might have on the **human body** and on the **planet** which are composed of **72%** of this basic element, water?

Emoto **demonstrates how much the consciousness of each of us contributes to creating and/or modifying the physical reality around us**.

Intentions, desires (which are vibrations not yet manifested), and what to say about words and sounds, can transform matter.

If you would like to learn more about this topic, I share some videos on the subject that you can view at the following links.

———————

Word search engine: Masaru Emoto

https://youtu.be/0ibiFfo6Qys

https://youtu.be/KeOsyl8xLdo

———————

We wish to extend this topic on the **power** of '**Word**' and '**Sounds**' by highlighting the **uniqueness** and **particularity** of the **Sanskrit language**.

Sanskrit is the language of the ancient Vedic civilization. A civilization that nowadays is associated with the geographical area of India, but which, according to various philosophical and historical texts, extended over almost the entire surface of the earth.

The Sanskrit language achieves an admirable **intrinsic relationship** between **sound** and **meaning**.

The Sanskrit language **harmoniously combines** '**Sound**' and '**Meaning**,' which **gives greater power** to the **conveyed meaning itself**.

In other words, this allows the '**meaning**' of a **word**, the **message**, to **penetrate** more **deeply** into the **human psyche** with greater **effects**.

To explain this concept, here is a practical example.

In Sanskrit to express the concept of '**Peace**' we use the word '**Shanti**,' which is derived from the root '**sham**,' meaning '**to calm**.'

The sound quality of the word '**Shanti**' is **peaceful**. On the other hand, the english word `**peace**' although it has the same basic meaning as 'Shanti,' has a **harsher sound quality** and, therefore, the sound associated with that word is not an optimal, or perfect, 'vehicle' for carrying its meaning.

You can do a personal test by **repeating** these two words, '**shanti**' and '**peace**,' for a few **minutes**. Finally you will be realising which one of the two words makes you feel more peaceful!

Of course, the meaning of the Thought, or Word, I want to convey is of fundamental importance. It is better to say something meaningful in an imperfect way than to say something insignificant in style!!!

Indeed, the ideal condition is for sound and meaning to be in harmony.

The sound 'reflects' the word and the meaning 'reflects' the mind.

It is important that the two, sound and meaning, resonate together with the same frequency. Thus our words will perfectly express what we want to convey and have the greatest effect and benefit on our listener.

This is the peculiarity of the Sanskrit language, which is considered the mother of all languages.

MANTRA

The Sanskrit term **MANTRA** is composed of two words, '**MAN**' and '**TRA**'.

The word '**MAN**' means '**Mind, Thought, Act of Thinking, Intellect, Breath, Living Soul.**'

While the word '**TRA**' means '**that Liberates, that Accomplishes, that Acts, that Protects, that Transforms.**'

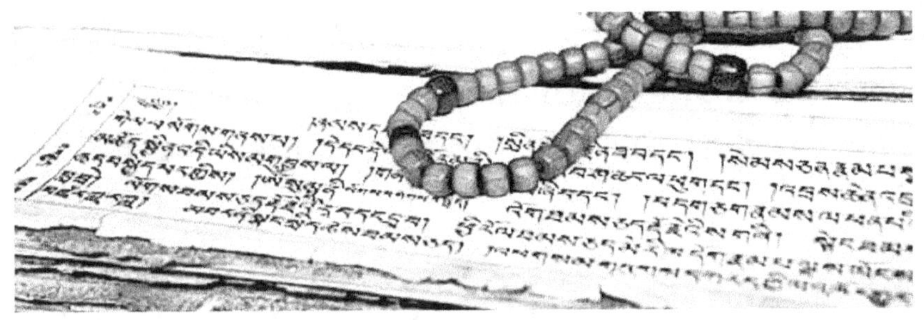

So put together the two words mean:

"**formula that frees the mind**" or "**tool that brings the mind from a state of continuous movement to one of calm and stillness**" or "**practice that protects our capacity to think**" or even "**formula that transforms our thoughts.**"

At a linguistic level, the Sanskrit word **MANTRA** implies a **specific structure of sound patterns, encoded in syllables and vowels**, which functions as a (spiritual) **tool** for **transforming** the **psychic state** of a human being from a state of **low knowledge** to a stage of **full knowledge** and **liberation.**

Sanskrit is a 'vibrational' **language**, so reciting mantras in Sanskrit creates a **sound vibration** that interacts with the human being on various levels: **physical, psychic** and **spiritual.**

The VEDIC MANTRA is a sacred formula, or expression, composed of a word or sequence of words.

If you wish to access its potential, it is important to understand the three elements that energetically activate the mantra itself (**Sound, Prana and Mind**).

- **'SOUND'ELEMENT**

The effect of a mantra depends first on **the energy inherent in the nature of its sound, the different qualities of the vowels and consonants recited, and the particularities of pronunciation.**

Each sound acts as a 'vehicle' and has a quality that reflects the potential meanings it carries. The **'Sound' element can be considered the 'physical body' of the Mantra.**

- ### 'PRANA' ELEMENT

The **effect** of a **mantra** depends on **how its sound is produced**. The same sound can be produced with more or less **force**, **intensity** and **speed**, which will naturally **alter** its **energy** and **impact**.

This is where the various types of tones and the precise way the mantra is handled through the breath come into play. **The 'Prana' element can be considered the 'life force' of the mantra.**

- ### 'MIND' ELEMENT

(Element 'Mind' or 'Attitude')

The effect of a mantra is influenced by the **thought, meaning, intention** and **emotion with which we utter the mantra.**

This element represents the 'Mind and Heart' of the mantra.

If in the **recitation** of the **MANTRA** we can **manage, harmonise and become aware of all three elements, then we gain full benefits.**

I emphasise that the benefits can be on a physical, psychic and/or spiritual level.

The VEDIC MANTRAs, in their highest sense, are **formulas** that allow us to **connect** to **our true inner essence**, to the **true nature of which we are a part of**: whether we then call it cosmic energy, Divinity, Universe, Absolute Truth or any other energetic aspect, initially is not essential.

The real essential aspect is that MANTRAs connect us with our deepest nature by acting directly on the unconscious.

We know very well that we cannot access the sphere of the **unconscious** with a conscious mind, so **MANTRAs** are an **invaluable tool**.

The MANTRA is yoga's main tool for controlling and calming the mind and managing the unconsciousness.

This state of **inner peace** is the **starting point** for accessing **higher understandings** of our **true spiritual nature**.

Meditation & Mantra

How can we understand, from a **partial** but **tangible scientific** point of view, the calming, relaxing and purifying effect of **Mantra recitation**?

I would like to introduce the concept of '**mindful meditation**'.

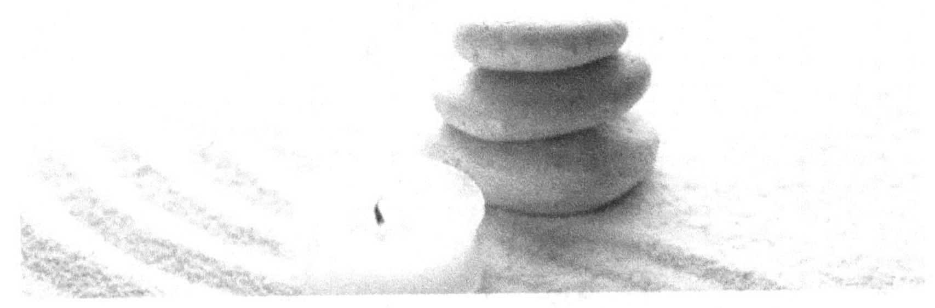

Meditating is a 'normal' process, in the norm, meaning it is a mental activity that every human being can perform, and often does, without even recognising that, in fact, he or she is meditating.

Meditating is not an esoteric activity, a religious act, but a '**psycho-biological**' and '**bio-energetic**' **process**. A process that is also used to create the preconditions for accessing higher levels of transcendence.

What happens to our brain when we enter a meditative state?

The brain is a very complex organ consisting of two hemispheres that are part of a reticular structure full of highly articulated connections.

The latest neurological research tools (functional magnetic resonance imaging, etc.), make it possible to show changes in brain activity and gain a deeper understanding of how the brain works by associating brain function with the activation of one or more areas of the brain, whether in the left or right hemisphere.

Thus, the dichotomous 'right hemisphere/left hemisphere' distinction (while valid), seems a bit too simplistic, incomplete and inaccurate.

Still I would ask you, for the **purpose of our analysis**, to adopt this **simplistic view** and be able to come to useful **conclusions** together for a better understanding of the topic '**Meditation**'.

Different areas of the brain have different functions. We have two hemispheres with different functions.

The left hemisphere is logical, sequential, analytical, rational and executive.

It also has a special feature, which is that it has a function of arranging events, objects, images in temporal sequence. It functions somewhat like a clock, that is, it makes us always aware of the passing of time.

Here is a list of its characteristics.

Left Hemisphere

Verbal: uses words, vocabulary, to name and define;

Analytical: analyses things and realities into their parts;

Symbolic: uses symbols and signs;

Abstract: from a detail represents reality in its entirety;

Temporal: arranges objects and events in temporal sequence;

Rational: arrives at well-founded conclusions based on reasoning;

Digital: uses the numerical method;

Logical: draws conclusions on logical principles;

Linear: thinks in sequential terms.

The right hemisphere has general holistic, intuitive, emotional, creative, musical and spiritual functions.

Above all, it does not know what the concept of time is.

Here is a list of its characteristics.

Right Hemisphere

Nonverbal: aware of reality but unable to describe it verbally;

Synthetic: unites the parts forming a whole;

Concrete: represents things as they are in the present moment;

Analogical: sees similarities, does not understand metaphorical relationships;

Timeless: without a sense of time;

Non-rational: does not require rational foundations of facts;

Spatial: perceives objects through their mutual spatial relationship, as parts of a whole;

Holistic: sees things as a whole, sometimes in contrast to the left hemisphere.

All these functions are available to each of us. We are all a bit like technicians who have a whole range of tools in their workshops in order to do their work. The more the technician is aware of the tools he has, the more he will use them!

At this point I ask, "Have you ever been hypnotised by the flame of a candle or bonfire on a night on the beach, completely forgetting the passage of time and everything around you?"

If the answer is "Yes," well then at that moment you had entered a meditative state.

Meditating consists of being able to direct the attention of the left hemisphere (or those areas that perform the logical, rational functions) **to a specific object in a conscious way**.

Said another way, we must succeed in the intent to partially deactivate all those abstract, logical, rational functions, characteristic of certain areas of the brain, which give continuous rise to the sequential analysis of intrusive thoughts. In short, we must reach a state in which the brain stops processing 'too actively' the information, the impressions it receives (both external and internal).

By doing so, the right hemisphere, which **has no temporal function**, can enter a **state of total isolation and evasion from surrounding reality and can become completely absorbed in a single object** (ecstasy). The meditative state is thus reached.

Various objects can be used to enter meditation.

In our case we use VEDIC MANTRAs, which have a special efficacy, as seen above. But objects such as a candle, a mandala, a bell, one's own breath can also be used.

The repetitive sequence of Mantra recitation is an action that engages the logical, temporal, rational function of the brain (left hemisphere), in focusing on that specific activity.

In this way, the holistic, timeless, synthetic, concrete functions of those areas of the brain assigned to such functions (right hemisphere) **can be fully expressed**, such as the flourishing and development of positive emotions and feelings.

In such a meditative process we come out of direct perception of time, space, and that whole sequence of intrusive thoughts other than our object of meditation. Then the power of the mantra, in terms of sound vibration, can manifest in its full intensity.

This is meditation with Mantra.

I want to emphasise that the intrinsic effect of mantra vibration on human beings takes effect regardless of whether they fully achieve a meditative state. Clearly if one can meditate optimally, the effect of the mantra is amplified.

Below I present a possible explanation of what happens in certain parts of the brain during meditation.

Frontal lobe

This is the most highly developed part of the brain, responsible for reasoning, planning, emotions and awareness. During meditation, the frontal cortex tends to reduce its activity.

Parietal lobe

This part of the brain processes sensory information about the surrounding world, giving orientation in time and space. During meditation, activity in the parietal lobe slows down.

Thalamus

This organ controls the senses and focuses our attention by allowing some sensory data to access areas deeper in the brain, while blocking others. Meditation reduces the flow of incoming information to this organ.

Reticular formation

This is the sentinel of the brain. This central nervous system structure receives incoming stimuli from outside and puts the brain on alert, ready to respond. Meditation causes the incoming arousal signal to be 'sent back to the sender' (please do not disturb!).

Based on all these considerations, we can only **imagine** how much **vital energy** remains **available** during **meditation**. All this energy is used by our body in order to be able to activate and support all those **purification processes** of the **physical** and the **psyche** (including the unconscious mind).

By accessing the following link you can listen to an example of guided meditation on breathing and on recitation of the mantra 'Om'.

https://youtu.be/
jWQcI5C6Wf0

https://youtu.be/jWQcI5C6Wf0

Mantra Yoga

Mantra Yoga is the practice of **union (yoga)** with the various aspects of the **Divine** through the **recitation** of **Vedic Mantras**.

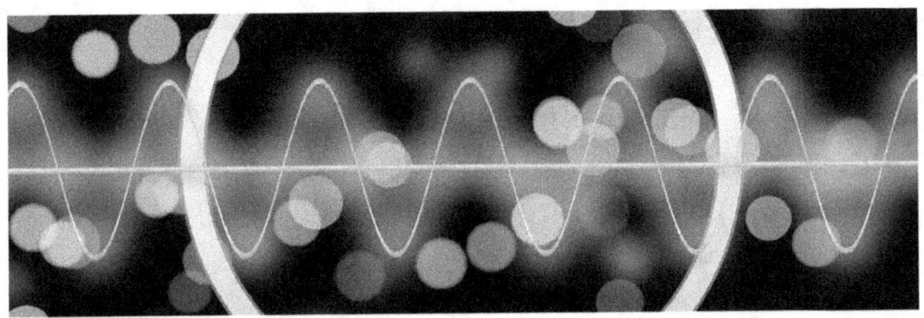

Mantra Yoga reflects, on an empirical, practical level, the entire 'Yoga of Sound' (Shabda Yoga), which formulates transcendental sound as the supreme reality of the universe.

Mantra Yoga is not a type of mantra, but the actual **process** for the **proper use** of the **sacred formulas** (the Mantras) that Vedic sages have handed down for millennia.

The practice of Mantra Yoga consists of reciting and listening (for a time) **to the chosen mantra** under specific **attitudinal** and **behavioural** **conditions** that enables us to **reach higher levels**

of **consciousness**, which we would not be able to **perceive under** 'normal' **conditions**.

During the practice of mantra-yoga I recommend that you gradually push your **meditation into complete concentration** on the **sound** (of the mantra) and rely on the recitation of the Mantra itself, trying to understand and 'make your own' its power and effects.

I am sure that through this combination of concentration, meditation and trust, the sound (the mantra) will lead you 'by the hand' through the various aspects of the Divine.

This progressive exercise will open new horizons for you about the origin of your own consciousness.

The Vedic mantra can equally be recited **aloud** or **whispered**, as the sound vibrations, penetrating directly into the unconscious, produce changes at the subliminal level.

The vibratory effect of Mantra recitation has the ability to induce a feeling of calmness in the mind. The mind becomes quiet, focused and reflective, allowing our **awareness** to **vibrate with the mantra itself**.

When you start vibrating the mantra, conditions are created for you to connect to the original transcendental sound, which is manifested through the mantra.

The effects of Mantra recitation practice can be magnified, enhanced, by combining, with the practice, the use of musical instruments (bhajana) and/or collective, harmonious recitation with other people (kirtana).

Collective chanting with musical instruments exploits the principle of synergistic and harmonic amplification of sound intensity and makes the effects of Mantra more effective.

To understand the concept of amplification, I can give you as an example a **pond of water** into which a **stone** is **thrown**.

Concentric waves will form on the surface of the water, propagating in all directions with a certain wave height.

If we throw more pebbles or heavier stones, at the same spot (to ensure the harmonic aspect), concentric waves of **increasing intensity** or **wave height** will be **created**.

This is the basic principle of collective chanting (kirtana)!

But what are the main purposes of Mantra Yoga?

- Developing Purity of Body and Mind

- Accessing Higher Levels of Consciousness

- In the next sections we will look at some of the best-known Mantras, including:

- the **primordial Mantra-seed (bija-mantra)** par excellence, the **Om** or **Omkara**;

- various **personal Mantras**, which are generally invocations of energies of nature, mind and spirit of a Deity or divine being.

Why 'Personal' Mantras?

Why do I place so much emphasis on PERSONAL MANTRAs? And especially why do I emphasise the aspect of knowing the Person 'behind the Mantra'?

We all have friends, relatives and acquaintances who, in one way or another, know parts of our character, personality, habits and tastes.

The more intimately they are connected with us, the more they know us!

And we sense the difference between being called by name by our close friend or a person not too close to us, then what to say of a stranger!

It's a whole different vibration! The timbre and tone of their voice awakens different emotions and feelings in us!

The same goes for the recitation of MANTRAs.

We can recite Mantras with different kinds of feelings and intentions, and this will vary the effect, depth and effectiveness of the MANTRA.

Many of the most common Mantras nowadays (not only the Vedic ones) are often recited in a 'non-personal' way, i.e., one pronounces the Mantra without, however, intending to enter into a deep relationship with the 'Person' the mantra represents.

Often this happens because no one has introduced us to the Person of the Mantra! I have found that, often, not even the 'guides' who try to give us information about the specific Mantra know or understand the personal aspect of it!

The consequence is that we aim directly at getting the benefit, the result of the Mantra, leaving the 'Person' aside.

I do not deny that even just chanting the Mantra will certainly bring about a result, but, in my experience, this will be partial, limited and, in the long run, not completely satisfying.

It is as if for business reasons we always go to eat at a small restaurant. Yes, we tastefully appreciate the quality of the food, but sooner or later we will try other places.

But if, on the other hand, we start to get to know the cook and a relationship of affection and friendship is created with her (him), we will be predisposed to keep going to that small restaurant and maybe, one day, the cook might even surprise us by cooking our favorite dish with affection and love!!!

At that point, in addition to forgetting to go out to lunch elsewhere, we will also feel very satisfied and happy with the new relationship.

I would like to share with you the following story that shows the importance of connecting with the 'Person' behind the Mantra, at least that is my personal experience.

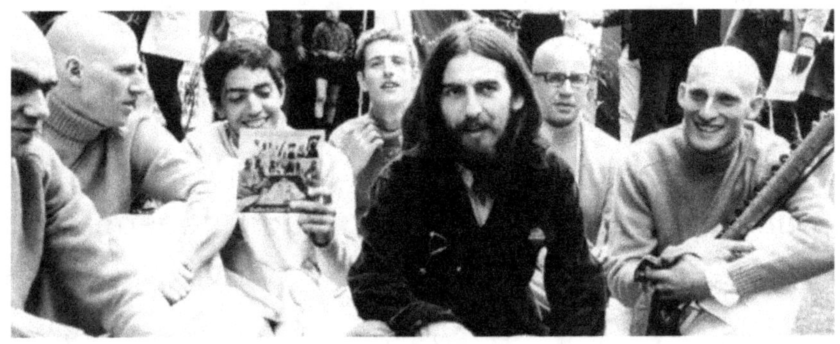

When I was younger, the song 'My sweet Lord' by George Harrison, former Beatles member, entered my list of most favourite songs. It was about the 1990s.

(At the end of the chapter I provide you with a link to the song in the spirit of sharing.)

I often listened to this song, which I quite liked for its musicality, although my English at that time was very poor and I did not grasp the full meaning of the lyrics.

However, the part that most intrigued me, but at the same time left me bewildered, was the refrain. A Mantra I had never heard, which I did not know and understand.

I sensed a certain mystical wave, but I could not define it, and although I liked it, in a short time it left me somewhat dissatisfied and therefore I stopped listening to such a song.

After a few years I met a person who had been on various spiritual paths, and one day it happened that we had the chance to listen to this song. I noticed that he appreciated the lyrics and even hummed the refrain with much feeling and pleasure. Then I took the opportunity to ask if he knew what it meant.

This spiritualist began to explain to me the meaning of the mantra (it was the Hare Krishna mantra!) and told me stories about Krishna and Rama, who They were, how They lived and what They represented.

From that day I listened to that song with a whole new predisposition and understanding, also developing feelings of appreciation and a renewed desire to understand more about those 'Persons'.

I won't hide from you that, over time, I also developed small and large personal and spiritual realisations.

That is why in this little guide-book I present a list of 'Personal Mantras' and their stories which will enable you to discover some aspects of the Persons 'behind the Mantra', some of their characteristics, qualities and peculiarities.

You will find that it is the most outstanding way to know and get incredible benefits from Mantras.

Link to the song 'My sweet Lord' by George Harrison.

https://youtu.be/B0Kh2yOCAJs

https://youtu.be/B0Kh2yOCAJs

Om - Omkara

The Mantra Om is considered the **primordial sound**, the initial vibration, from which all the **Universe originated**. We will analyse this mantra only on a cognitive level, as it has a function of **invocation**.

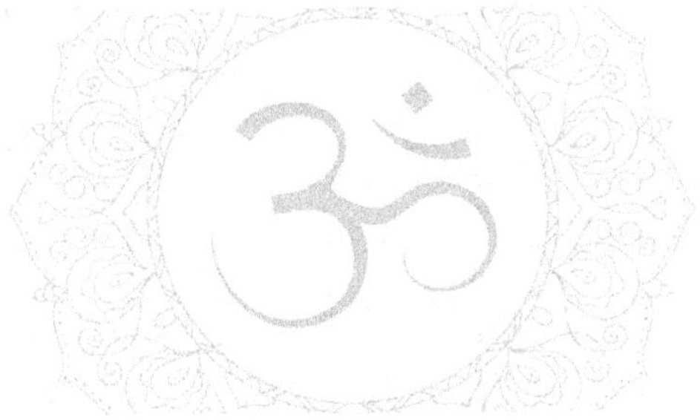

The Mantra **Om** is the quintessential mantra, a 'bija-mantra,' or 'mantra-seed,' a very **concise formula** that is inserted at the beginning of virtually all Vedic mantras as an **invocation** of the **Supreme**.

In Vedic culture, spiritualists, who undertake the performance of sacrifices, charity and penances according to the rules of the scriptures, always **begin** their **practices** by **uttering Om** in order to **reach** the **Supreme**.

According to the Yogic science of Mantra, there are four types of sound waves: (1) standing waves, (2) reverberating waves, (3) oscillating waves and (4) transcendental waves.

Om is the harmonic union of these waves.

To understand this aspect we can see the letter Om as the set of the letters A, U, M.

The emission of "A" creates the standing waves, those of "U" and "M" the reverberating and oscillating waves, respectively. Finally, the meditation of the Om at the heart center creates the transcendental waves.

According to the Vedic scriptures (Padma Purana), the transcendental mantra Om includes:

The letter 'A,' which represents the source of all creative energies (the Creator);

The letter 'U', which represents spiritual and material energy (the Creation);

The letter 'M,' representing individual energy (the Creatures).

'Om' allows the ascent and expansion of energy. It **carries** the **sound vibration** through the **body's** main **energy points (chakras)** up to the top of the head.

It enables us to find **harmony** with the **forces** of the **universe**, both **inwardly** and **outwardly**. It attunes us to **cosmic reality** and its sacred vibrations.

'Om' has the ability to prepare and clear the mind for meditation on the Divine.

I mentioned earlier that Mantras have effects at various energetic levels: physical, psychic and spiritual.

Let us look at them together.

Effects on the Physical Body

Helps purify the body

Meditation with the mantra Om helps regulate blood circulation and provide more oxygen supply in the body. This process, which includes deep and constant breathing, promotes the elimination of toxins. Sages claim that it enables one to maintain a state of inner and outer youthfulness.

Helps the heart and digestive system

In addition to regulating blood flow, the repetition of the Om sound also helps **regulate blood pressure**. When we temporarily detach ourselves from the worries of the world, the heartbeat and breathing return to normal levels. The vibrations caused by the Om and deep breathing also strengthen the **digestive system**.

Stimulates self-control

The human psyche is continuously subjected to strong impulses or drives (tongue, anger, stomach, genitals, etc.), and it is very difficult to control strong feelings and emotions such as frustration, anger, irritation and sadness.

Sometimes, thus urged, we react aggressively for unnecessary reasons, which we later regret. I think it's a dynamic that we all share. What do you think?

The mantra Om **strengthens** the **will, mind** and **consciousness**.

This allows us to calmly analyse situations and find a logical, non-impulsive, solution to the problem.

When we are more aware of our feelings and emotions we can develop greater sensitivity towards other people.

Helps reduce stress

As analysed in the section 'Mantra and Meditation' recitation of the mantra Om interacts with our brain, reducing the production of adrenaline which in turn reduces stress.

It helps us to think positively

When we experience fatigue or inability to focus on work, the daily practice of Om recitation increases the level of endorphins that promote a sense of freshness and relaxation.

In addition, endorphins balance hormone secretion, which plays a significant role in mood swings.

By chanting the mantra Om you are asking to activate a purification of mind, body and spirit, and to be able to receive a higher intellect for spiritual success in your life.

Below I provide a link to listen to a very deep recitation of the mantra Om.

https://youtu.be/4usQ20n1ZKk

https://youtu.be/4usQ20n1ZKk

Om Namah Shivaya

Om - Bija invocation mantra

Namah - is the mantra of reverence and surrender and means 'my respects and obeisances.' It is used to honour and surrender to the Deity who is glorified in the Mantra

Shivaya - Shiva is one of the three main deities in Vedic tradition. He is the deity responsible for the destruction of the universe. The suffix -ya means 'to you'

The Mantra **'Om namah Shivaya'** means **'My respects to you, Lord Shiva'** or **'I surrender myself to you, Lord Shiva'**. The primordial syllable 'Om' enhances the effects of the mantra.

Spiritual benefits

The mantra 'Om Namah Shivaya' is first encountered in the hymn 'Rudram' of the Yajur Veda. Such a mantra grants knowledge of that which is eternal.

This Mantra consists of five syllables that are connected to:

- the five primary elements of this universe: ether, air, fire, water, earth;

- the five senses of human being;

- the five types of air (prana);

- five of seven energy centres (chakras) of the body.

Each primary element is connected to a sensory organ of action.

Repetition of the mantra purifies all the above elements, which contributes to outer and inner transformation.

According to the Vedic conception of material creation, the Universe is subject to continuous transformation: it is created, it is maintained for a time and then it is destroyed. This is an **eternal** and **cyclical** process. Shiva is the divine manifestation that performs the cosmic function of destroying the Universe.

If we transfer this understanding from the macrocosm to the microcosm, the inner dimension of man, we understand how **Shiva** can be the '**tool**' that helps us 'destroy,' **overcome**, our 'old' **visions** and **limitations**, to make way for **new** prosperous **realities**.

Physical benefits

'Om Namah Shivaya' is a solar Mantra, 'dynamic' in nature. In relation to the way it is performed, its recitation is indicated for curing different kinds of diseases.

Psychic benefits

The Mantra can be performed at different 'levels'; one level is that used by the advanced practitioner to bring about a quick awakening of the psychic force.

Recitation of the mantra 'Om Namah Shivaya', with faith and awareness of its meaning, **eliminates despair, envy, anger, greed, removes illusions, and frees the person from existing mental impurity.**

The mantra transforms a person's consciousness and his or her own life, **brings peace**, **happiness**, **prosperity** and a sense of **unity** with the **whole world**.

To understand why one can develop all these physical and mental benefits, one must know, understand and appreciate Lord Shiva and his extraordinary qualities. Therefore, I narrate you the following story.

History of the churning of the cosmic ocean

The history of the universe is characterised by a constant search for balance between 'forces of light' and 'forces of darkness', both at the level of microcosm and macrocosm.

Due to a series of special conditions, the celestial beings lost their kingdom, defeated by the beings of darkness.

Their only purpose in life was to regain their position of control. They were advised to enter into a peace pact with the forces of darkness. In this way they would cooperate with them in order to obtain the nectar of immortality (amrita) and with this be able to regain their kingdom.

But in order to obtain this 'elixir of long life' they had to perform a tremendous, almost impossible task, namely to churn the cosmic ocean, from which the elixir itself would be produced.

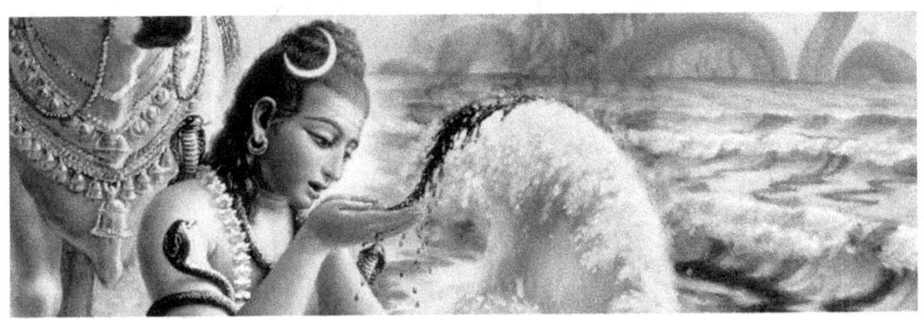

Clearly both sides secretly thought, once they obtained the elixir, they would overpower their opponents and drink the elixir first.

To accomplish the feat they used, as a staff, a giant mountain (Mandara) and plunged it into the ocean by resting it on a giant turtle (Kurma).

Once they rested the mountain on the turtle, the King of Serpents, an enormous snake (Vasuki Nagaraja) made himself available to serve as a rope, which they twisted around the Mandara mountain.

The celestial beings grabbed it from the side of the tail, while the eternal rivals grabbed it from the side of the multiple mouths and, all together, began to pull it to one side and the other, causing the mountain to rotate on itself and thus churning the cosmic ocean from which gigantic waves rose.

By dint of churning the ocean, a terrible poison (halakuta) began to form, which began to destroy everything it touched.

Both the celestial beings and the being of darkness realised that the situation had become very serious. The total destruction of the universe itself was threatened.

Therefore they all went to the place where Shiva dwelt and asked him for his quick intervention.

After receiving prayers for help from all living beings, Shiva agreed to drink the destructive poison.

He therefore picked it up, taking it in the palm of his hand, and swallowed it. As soon as Shiva drank the poison, his neck turned blue. This is why Shiva is also called Nilakantha, meaning 'with a blue throat'.

From this story we can understand the power, compassion and benevolence of Lord Shiva.

By chanting this mantra you aspire to develop the luminous qualities of Lord Shiva, as well as gain all the benefits mentioned above.

Chanting the mantra you could also ask Lord Shiva to remove attitudinal and behavioral 'poisons' from your heart: envy, jealousy, hatred, depression, malice, anger, etc.

To end the short story, the heavenly beings finally succeeded in obtaining and drinking the elixir of immortality first and regained their kingdom.

Below I provide a link to listen to a sound version of this mantra.

https://youtu.be/SsZYhhFxZrY

https://youtu.be/SsZYhhFxZrY

Om Namo Narayanaya

Om - Bija invocation mantra

Namo - is the mantra of reverence and surrender and means 'my respects and obeisances'. It is used to honour and surrender to the Deity who is glorified in the Mantra

Narayanaya - Narayana is a divine manifestation of the Absolute Truth. The term 'Nara' means 'human being' while the term 'ayana' means 'one who grants protection'

The mantra '**Om Namo Narayanaya**' means:

'**My respects to you, Lord Narayana, who grant protection to all human beings'**.

In addition to protection, the mantra '**Om Namo Narayanaya**' bestows **love**, **strength**, **glory**, **wisdom**, **liberation** and the **ability** to **overcome obstacles arising** from **selfishness** and **ignorance**.

This is one of the main mantras used to repeat the name of the Divine and glorify the power of the Divine. Repeating this mantra **creates spiritual merits** and the **Supreme** will also **take care** of our **material well-being**.

Chanting this mantra **decreases** the **influence, impulse** and **drives** of the **mind**, and allows us to access a **state** of **mind** of **divine grace**.

Since it is a protection mantra, it enables you to **keep** in **balance** or **rebalance** the **energies** of your **physical body** and thus ensure **health** and **longevity**.

To understand the importance and mercy of this Mantra I will tell you the story of Ajamila.

Story of Ajamila

Ajamila had been brought up by his parents as a perfect scholar (brahmana).

One day young Ajamila was walking in the forest on his way home. Unexpectedly he saw some movement in the vegetation and realised that it was the amorous effusions between a man and a woman.

This happening brought back into his consciousness various unconscious material desires. Gradually his mental condition changed to such an extent that he began to desire the company of the very woman he had seen in the forest.

Ajamila abandoned his family and young wife and became a great thief, murderer, and swindler. He began to engage in numerous ungodly activities in order to satisfy his greed and his new companion.

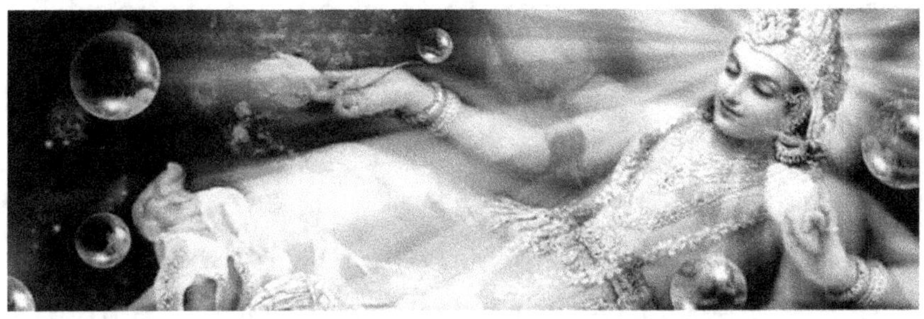

Ajamila had ten children with this woman, the last of whom was named Narayana, who was conceived when Ajamila was already of advanced age.

Ajamila became very old and the time of death came for him. According to Vedic tradition when a very ungodly person is about to die, terrifying beings, the servants of the Lord of Death, manifest themselves.

And these beings showed up punctually at Ajamila's deathbed in order to catch him and take him to hell.

Ajamila, who was very attached to his youngest son, in fear cried out in great desperation, seeking help, the name of his little son Narayana.

At that point beings of celestial form appeared and rescued Ajamila and granted him the chance to redeem himself and resume his spiritual path.

This last event demonstrates the power of reciting the name Narayana, although, as in this story, there was no real intention to seek protection from the Supreme Person.

From this story we can understand the power of the name Narayana which (1) protects from all difficult situations in life, even the most hopeless, (2) eliminates all reactions of our ungodly activities and (3) grants the right consciousness to resume or deepen our spiritual life.

By chanting this mantra you can ask the Supreme for protection in every aspect of your life and the strength to embark on or persevere in the path of spiritual fulfilment.

Returning to Ajamila's story, there is a happy ending. He had the opportunity to live a few more years. And he immediately took advantage of it traveling to a holy place and achieve spiritual perfection.

Below I share a link to listen to a sound version of this mantra.

https://youtu.be/y5IdVbqjkrE

https://youtu.be/y5IdVbqjkrE

Om Namo Bhagavate Vasudevaya

Om - Bija invocation mantra

Namo-it is the mantra of reverence and surrender and means 'my respects and obeisances'

Bhagavate - It is the Absolute Truth or the all-pervading Supreme Being

Vasudevaya - He is the Absolute Truth who fully manages all His energies. In the Vedic tradition He is Lord Krishna

The mantra **'Om Namo Bhagavate Vasudevaya'** means, in general, **'I offer my homages to the Supreme Person who resides everywhere in full awareness and in full control of all His energies'**, and, in a more personal way, **'I offer my** respectful obeisances to the son of Vasudeva (Krishna), the Supreme Person'.

It is a sacred mantra of enormous power.

The effect of this mantra is such that **it can provide you with invaluable spiritual support in order to achieve liberation from the difficulties and sufferings** of this material dimension.

In addition, many Vedic texts clearly and seriously state that chanting this mantra has the power to neutralise all ungodly activities committed unconsciously.

The Mantra **'Om Namo Bhagavate Vasudevaya'** **keeps all negative energies away**. It **creates** an **invisible** and **invincible shield around you**. A shield that allows only positive and divine energies to pass through.

To understand the importance and mercy of this Mantra I tell you the story of Gajendra.

Story of the elephant Gajendra

In the middle of the cosmic ocean there is a wonderful and imposing mountain known as Trikuta.

In one of the valleys of Trikuta mountain there is a beautiful garden known by the name of Rtumat, which was created by the celestial being of water (Varuna), and in that area there is a wonderful lake.

One day Gajendra the child of the elephants, in order to have fun together with his companions, went to bathe in this lake and thereby disturbed the inhabitants of those waters.

The chief of the crocodiles of that lake, who was very powerful, became very disturbed and immediately attacked the elephant by biting him in the leg.

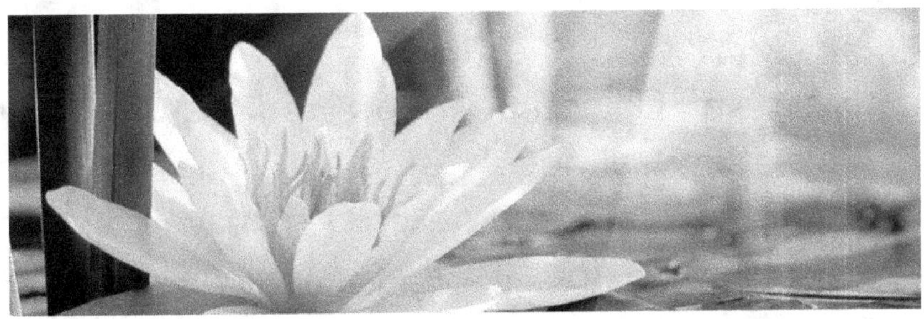

The strenuous struggle that followed went on for a thousand years. The elephant began to lose its mental, physical and sensory strength.

In contrast, the crocodile, which is an aquatic animal, saw its enthusiasm, physical strength and sensory power increase.

The king of the elephants understood that he was in a desperate condition and that no one, neither his friends nor his family, could save him from danger. Then he was seized with the fear of death.

After mature reflection he finally came to the following decision, "The other elephants, who are my friends and relatives, could not save me from this danger. What then can my wives do? They cannot do anything. By the will of providence I have been attacked by this crocodile, so I will seek refuge in the Supreme Person, Who is always the refuge of all. I submit myself to Him, the great and powerful Supreme Authority, who is the true refuge of every being".

At that point Gajendra picked up a lotus flower with his trunk, although in great suffering, and dedicated to the Supreme Lord a prayer he had learned in his previous life that began with the very mantra **'Om namo bhagavate vasudevaya'**.

The results were incredible. Gajendra received full protection from the Supreme Lord, was saved from that situation and resumed his normal life but with a renewed spiritual consciousness.

By chanting this mantra you can ask the Divine to 'awaken' your spiritual awareness, protect

your spiritual desires and remove all those inner qualities deleterious to the attainment of true ultimate happiness.

Below I share a link to listen to a sound version of this mantra.

https://youtu.be/
3blvsxheLgo

https://youtu.be/3blvsxheLgo

Jaya Sita Rama

Jaya - Sanskrit word for 'Glory' or 'victory'

Sita - Energy of Compassion and Energy of Love. Eternal companion of Rama (Ramachandra)

Rama - Divine Manifestation. The term means 'Source of all happiness'

The mantra **'Jaya Sita Rama'** means **'Glory to Sita and Ramachandra, the energies of Love and Bliss'**.

Sita and Ramachandra represent, besides being Divine manifestations, those people who act or have acted as our references in various spheres of our lives-such as family, education, spirituality, etc.

By reciting the mantra **'Jaya Sita Rama' you are expressing a feeling of gratitude, recognition and thanks, for all that you are and have achieved in life**.

These sentiments are primarily addressed to Divine energies, but also to parents, family members, friends, teachers and spiritual guides.

Rama symbolises the **inner fervour** in the energy center (chakra) of the **solar plexus** (manipura) that **purifies** the **body** and **spirit**.

Sita symbolises the **energy** in the **basal energy center** (muladhara chakra) that gives **stability** and **calms** the **mind**.

Through the recitation of the mantra 'Jaya Sita Rama' **the functions of the two hemispheres of the brain are balanced**.

It is also believed to **improve health** by **removing impurities** from the **body** and **mind** and to **promote** the **development** of **self-awareness**.

By chanting this mantra you are invoking the divine qualities of the **divine couple, Sita** and **Rama**.

To understand the qualities, character, strength and stature of these divine figures, Ramachandra

and Sita, I tell you this story from the Ramayana
(the story of their lives).

The meeting between Sita and Ramachandra

Sita was a young princess, the daughter of King
Janaka who ruled the kingdom of Mitila.

When Sita was still a child she often played with a
ball in the company of her friends. One day, while
they were all playing together, the ball ended up
under the structure on which rested the famous,
legendary 'arch of Shiva,' which had been given to
the king of Mithila.

Such was the situation that to access the lower
part of the structure and get the ball, Sita would
have to lift the arch itself.

Without even lingering and with much innocence,
Sita lifted the bow with her left hand and retrieved
the ball with the other.

When the royal guards, placed to guard the bow,
saw this scene, they immediately fainted. What
had happened?

The soldiers had been totally astonished and
stunned, as it usually took at least 5,000 warriors to
raise and move such a mystical bow. We can
imagine the power of Sita who lifted it without any

strain. For we know that Sita represents the Lord's inner and spiritual energy.

The soldiers reported the incident to King Janaka (Sita's father) who understood the nature and power of his daughter, so he decided that anyone who wanted to marry Sita would have to raise the bow at least once in his life. This became an inescapable and obligatory condition to marry her.

Given Sita's exceptional qualities and beauty, so many kings and princes of the world came to King Janaka's kingdom to try to raise the bow. But whatever their strength and sincere effort, no one ever succeeded in raising the legendary 'bow of Shiva,' not even by a millimeter!

After many years Prince Ramachandra, with his brother Lakshmana, came to Mitila, the capital of King Janaka's kingdom.

On that occasion he was traveling together with his spiritual master Vishvamitra.

As soon as the three outsiders entered the city, everyone understood that Ramachandra would accomplish the feat of raising the bow.

The next day King Janaka invited Ramachandra and Lakshmana to court and he arranged for Shiva's bow to be brought in.

To carry the bow from where it was to the royal palace it took 500 bulls pulling the chariot on which the bow rested and 5,000 men pushing it from behind.

Ramachandra, as soon as he saw the arch, asked the master if he could view it up close. The master agreed.

Ramachandra walked toward the arch with such confidence and assurance that he resembled the gait of a lion. Lord Ramachandra's manner of movement represented the moving qualities of five animals: the solemnity and confidence of the lion, the majesty of the elephant, the fury of the tiger, the fierceness of the bull, and the speed of the serpent.

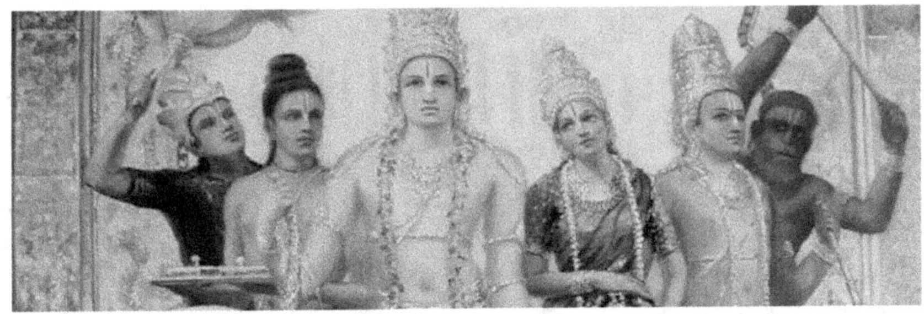

When he reached the bow, he circled around it with great respect three times. Then he asked the master if he could touch the bow. The master agreed. Then he asked him if he could lift it. The master again consented.

At that point Ramachandra lifted the bow without any effort, just as an adult male elephant lifts a lotus flower.

Finally he placed the bow on the ground and tried to put on the string. Abruptly the bow broke with a roar so loud that it was heard throughout the universe.

King Janaka began to dance with joy because he realised that Ramachandra had lifted the bow. He immediately asked Sita to get ready and handed her a garland to offer to Ramachandra that indicated the future wedding ceremony.

When Sita handed him the garland Rama said, "But I cannot marry you. If My father does not give me permission I cannot get married!"

King Janaka became very sad on hearing this.

Imagine how he felt. Thousands of people had tried to raise the bow, and the only one who had succeeded could not marry. Moreover, the bow had been broken. King Janaka was in despair. But Vishvamitra reassured him and said, "Rama did not say that he does not want to marry, but that he cannot unless he has his father's consent".

Now let us analyse how Sita felt. She had waited so many years for the right person. Now she had found him, but she could not get married. Any other girl would have fallen into depression.

Instead, Sita was very pleased with Ramachandra's response. I would like to point out Sita's unparalleled intelligence and ability to understand psychological aspects based on a simple answer from Ramachandra. Besides being a beautiful woman, she had exceptional intelligence, education, insight and vision.

Returning to the story, Sita had always thought that if she had a would-be groom, this person should manifest three important qualities.

The first quality was to have the strength to protect her in any situation (in fact, Ramachandra lifted the bow).

Second quality, even more important, was the man's ability to be able to clearly explain what was in his heart. When Sita heard the answer, the words, of Ramachandra, she knew that this was the right person, who could express himself clearly, directly, without delay.

Third quality was the ability to control the senses. Sita was a woman of immaculate qualities and incomparable beauty. Thousands of kings and princes had fought among themselves to marry her. And now Ramachandra, obedient to his social and family duties, said he could not marry her.

Anyway, King Dasharatha, Ramachandra's father, was informed about the incident and agreed to the marriage between Sita and Ramachandra.

From this short story we can understand the incredible qualities of the perfect gentleman in Rama and the perfect gentlewoman in Sita.

By reciting this mantra with knowledge, respect and admiration you can receive the blessings to be able to develop the incredible divine and spiritual qualities of Sita and Rama. In addition you can ask to develop in you the right ethical and moral behaviour towards society, friends, family members and all living beings.

Below is a link for you to listen to a sound version of this mantra.

https://youtu.be/
eGcxZz_aolE

https://youtu.be/eGcxZz_aolE

Jaya Radhe Govinda

Jaya - Sanskrit word for 'Glory' or 'Victory'

Radhe - Energy of Compassion and Energy of Love. Goddess of the Universe. Beloved of Krishna. Radhe is the vocative case of Radha

Govinda - Divine Manifestation. The term means the one who is 'the Lord of the senses of all human beings'

The mantra **'Jaya Radha Govinda'** means **'Glories to Radha and Govinda'** or **'Glories to the Energy of Compassion and Love of the Universe and to the Energy that governs the senses of all human beings'**.

From a spiritual point of view **Radha** is the **personification** of **Divine Love**. She is the internal, direct, primary energy of the Divine representing pure Compassion, Affection and Love.

Radha brings Joy and **Bliss** to the Divine (represented by Govinda, Krishna) and **to all living beings**. She is the one who enables the act of spiritual union between the individual soul and the Supreme soul (Govinda).

Radha is the receptacle of all divine and transcendental qualities.

When you chant the mantra **'Jaya Radhe Govinda'** you **connect** with **spiritual energy** and **acquire** its **qualities**.

The affection, love and compassion we exchange with other living beings testify to the health of our inner energy flow.

When you listen to the mantra **'Jaya Radhe Govinda'** your **'heart'**, the center of love, will **receive invigorating energy** achieving these benefits: (1) **improvement** of **relationships** in the **interpersonal sphere**, (2) **harmonisation** of the **inner world**, and (3) **awakening** of **positive qualities**.

When you chant or listen to this mantra with deep love, **Govinda**, the Lord of Senses, will **grant you** full **joy**, **love**, **courage** and **bliss**.

To understand the true relationship of affection and love between Radha and Govinda (Krishna), I will narrate you the following story.

Govinda's (Krishna) headache

I would like to make a small preface so as not to misunderstand the spiritual depth of this story. Govinda (Krishna), according to Vedic tradition, is the Absolute Truth, the Supreme Lord, totally independent. In other words, he can do what he wishes, when and how he wishes.

Govinda was lying on the bed and did not want to move. He was complaining of a very severe headache!!!

All the acquaintances, friends, and family members were puzzled. Such a situation had never been seen before.

That same day the great sage Narada Muni arrived in the city of Dwaraka and was immediately taken to the royal palace where Govinda was. Everyone knew that if anyone could solve the situation, find a remedy for Govinda's illness, that was the great sage.

Narada entered Govinda's quarters to visit him and stayed there for some time. All the courtiers and citizens were anxiously waiting, almost holding their breath.

When Narada came out of the room he had a determined walk, but on his face a small smile showed, well hidden.

Narada said, "Govinda has a headache. It seems that the only medicine is to sprinkle His head with the dust of the feet of those who truly love Him".

All the people present were very confused. How is this possible? Putting the dust of devotees' feet on the Lord's head? This is unheard of!!!

Narada began to approach everyone in the kingdom asking for some of the dust of their feet. But they all replied that it was impossible. Putting the dust of the feet on Govinda's head was like putting one's own feet there, and that was a total disrespect, with the clear risk of a rebirth in hell!

Finding no one, Narada headed for the village where Govinda had spent his childhood (Vrindavana) and where people who had great affection for Him still lived.

There Narada immediately met Radha, who had always had enormous affection and Love for Govinda.

The shepherdess walked very gracefully down a country path, carrying a jar full of milk with one hand, while her other hand lifted the edge of her skirt so as not to soil it with mud puddles.

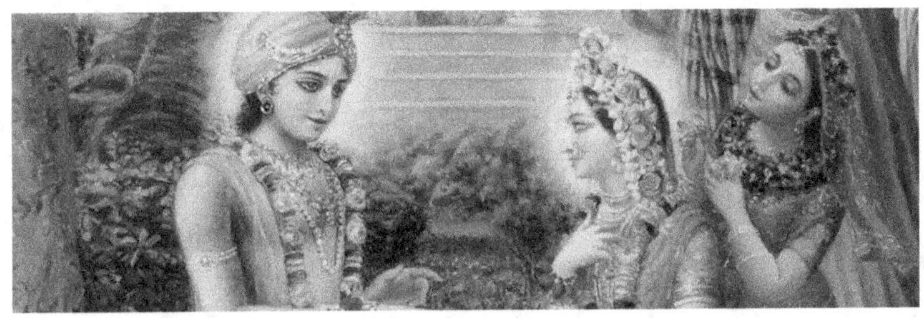

As soon as Radha saw the sage, she placed the vase at his feet and bowed respectfully.

Narada told her the story of Govinda's headache, and Radha grew paler and paler and almost fainted listening to her beloved's condition. Radha exclaimed with great concern, "There must be a cure!"

Narada paused and said, "The only cure is that the dust of the feet of those who love Him should be placed on His forehead. Only then will His headache end".

An expression of relief appeared on Radha's face and a resplendent smile graced it.

"That's it! Here, take this!" Sri Radha bent down and picked up the dust, made muddy by the rain, from one of the footprints he had left on the ground. She placed it on a plate and handed it with both hands to Narada Muni, saying: "Please take this, oh sage, and cure my beloved Govinda's headache".

At that point Narada looked at her with a doubtful look. "If you give me this powder, then there is a great possibility that you will go to hell in the next life".

Radha looked confused. "My dear Narada, why are you hesitating? My Lord is suffering".

Narada was shocked by Radha's determination. "Aren't you afraid of going to hell, my dear girl?"

But Radha replied: "It doesn't matter. I would be happy to live in hell if it would ease the suffering of my beloved Lord".

Narada immediately returned to the city of Dwaraka and put the powder from Radha's feet on Govinda's forehead, who got immediate relief from the headache.

This is the nature of Radha's unconditional divine love for Govinda. She would do anything to ensure eternal and continuous happiness for her beloved.

By chanting this mantra you could ask the Divine to make you develop love, strength and compassion in all your interpersonal relationships (marital, family, friendship).

Here is a link to listen to a sound version of this mantra.

https://youtu.be/AqA6YaMhpCE

https://youtu.be/AqA6YaMhpCE

Maha-Mantra

Hare - Energy of Compassion and Love energy

Krishna - Divine Manifestation. The term means 'Sublime Fascination' or 'He who is infinitely fascinating'

Rama - Divine Manifestation. The term means 'Source of all pleasure'

HARE KRISHNA HARE KRISHNA

KRISHNA KRISHNA HARE HARE

HARE RAMA HARE RAMA

RAMA RAMA HARE HARE

The **maha-mantra** (the great mantra) **Hare Krishna** is a very ancient mantra consisting of sixteen words and is found **mentioned** in the **Upanishads** (**kali-santarana Upanishad**).

The mantra consists of three words that are repeated in a specific order.

The deep meanings of the words and why the particular succession of such are very esoteric arguments that require special investigation. In this brief text I limit myself to some of the meanings.

First of all, the three names that are repeated in the maha-mantra are: **Hare**, **Krishna** and **Rama**.

These are names that invoke the **Absolute Reality** and in particular **His personal aspect**.

Hare is the **energy** of **Compassion**, it is the **energy** of **Love**, the sublime feeling we want to develop in our heart.

Krishna is the **Source** of **Sublime Charm**, the Supreme Person.

Rama is the divine manifestation that is the **Source** of **all pleasure**, of everything that satisfies us.

In the maha-mantra it is said that everything is present, precisely because there is Love and the Object of Love.

By reciting and chanting it you recognise your desire to manifest pure Love and Compassion.

Chanting the 'Maha Mantra' is a request to the Divine to become instruments of Love in the family, in society, in every interpersonal relationship.

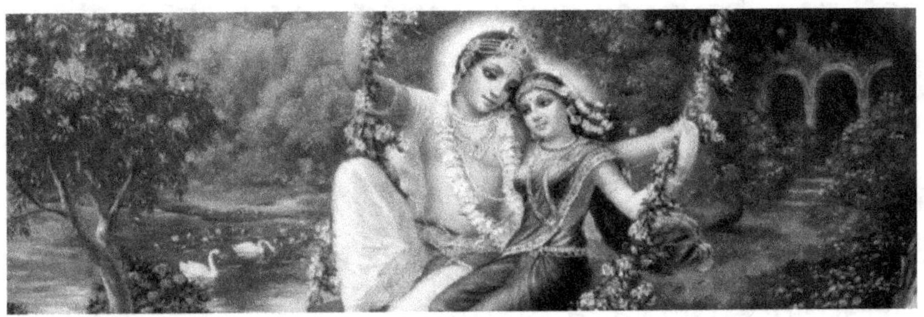

Recitation of this thousand-year-old mantra **enables you to fulfil all your desires and achieve many spiritual benefits.**

The **Hare Krishna mantra** has the power to **calm** and **control the mind and transform all kinds of mental disorders.** It enables you to perceive the essential spiritual quality in all your experiences in life.

The **maha-mantra purifies** the **heart** from **illusions, misunderstandings** and **anxieties** and is one of the few mantras that allows you to **remove** all the **reactions** of your **ungodly activities** (it **changes** your **destiny**).

Systematic recitation enables you to **develop knowledge, emotional detachment from the most difficult situations you experience in life** and can grant you liberation from the sense of suffering inherent in material existence.

The chanting of the maha-mantra will lead you to **develop** all **those virtuous** and **divine qualities** that you have always **longed for** and that will **improve** all the **interpersonal relationships** you have in place, so as to benefit not only **yourself**, but all the **people around you**.

The following story gives you an insight into the importance of maha-mantra.

The Great Blessing

Once upon a time there was a poor brahmana who worshipped Shiva in order to obtain a great blessing. Shiva reciprocated by advising his devotee to visit a great sage, Sanatana Gosvami.

So the brahmana went to the sage and informed him that Shiva had advised him to request the greatest blessing.

Sanatana Gosvami had a philosopher's stone that he kept together with the garbage. Following the request he gave the philosopher's stone to the poor brahmana, who was very happy to have it: simply by bringing iron into contact with the philosopher's stone he could obtain all the gold he desired.

After taking leave of the sage, the brahmana thought: "If the philosopher's stone is the greatest blessing, why did Sanatana Gosvami keep it near the garbage?"

So he went back and asked Sanatana Gosvami: "Sir, if this is the greatest blessing, why did you keep it near the garbage?"

Sanatana Gosvami replied. "Actually this is not the greatest blessing. But are you ready to receive the greatest blessing from me? Are you willing to give up material happiness for something that will give you inner satisfaction forever?"

The brahmana said: "Yes, Lord. Shiva has sent me to you to obtain the greatest blessing".

Then Sanatana Gosvami asked him to go and throw the philosopher's stone into the nearby river and return to him.

The poor brahmana obeyed, and upon his return Sanatana Gosvami initiated him in the chanting of the maha-mantra Hare Krishna. Thus, thanks to Shiva's blessing, the brahmana obtained the company of Krishna's greatest devotee and was initiated into the chanting of the maha-mantra, which granted him unimaginable happiness and inner bliss and a safe refuge even in those conditions and situations of life in which even owning a mountain of gold would be of no relief.

By chanting this mantra you ask for blessings for a sudden purification of body and spirit, to be serious and resolute in your spiritual quest and to become a true instrument of Love and Compassion.

You can recite or chant the maha-mantra at any moment of the day, individually or in a group.

In this way your every moment will be a gradual ascent to material and spiritual perfection.

Here is a link to listen to an audio version of this mantra.

https://youtu.be/q6AFDMKjJCQ

https://youtu.be/q6AFDMKjJCQ

Conclusions

Every human being is in search of **peace**, **happiness** and **freedom**. This **quest** is the main **goal** of **life** and is the **real challenge** of **human existence**.

Only a completely **peaceful** person hasn't anymore **stringent demands**, he is not **influenced** by the **consequences** of his **activities** and he is **truly self-sufficient**.

It is possible to find this **condition** of **inner peace through** the **recitation** or **chanting** of **Vedic MANTRAs**, as seen in the previous sections.

A constant **commitment** to Mantra-yoga practice is the '**key**' to being able to **take refuge** in **Mantras** and gain **protection** from the **Person** who is **glorified** in the **Mantra** itself.

But I do not believe in miracles (except as exceptional events). **Enthusiasm**, **patience** and **trust** are the inner states that give us **access** to the Mantra and to that **personal relationship** that will **grant us material** and, above all, **spiritual benefits**.

Mantra is that friend who will grant us peace and tranquility. But to recognise whether a person can be a friend, we need to **invest time** in hanging out with him and **getting** to **know** him more and more.

If his qualities, his character prove to be pleasant, divine and sublime, we will surely accept him as a friend, the best friend.

The secret of success is to create a personal relationship with the Mantra.

Truly hoping that you have enjoyed this little book, I wish you much inspiration in beginning, or continuing with more depth, the practice of Mantra recitation and invite you to learn more deeply about the Vedic philosophy and the divine people we have presented in this booklet.

I would also be very grateful to receive your feedback, questions, comments, requests for clarification and/or further investigation of specific topics related to the theme of this little book. Please feel free to use our email:

educazionevedica@gmail.com